ROSEMARIE PARSE

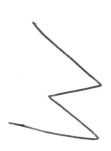

Notes on Nursing Theories

SERIES EDITORS
Chris Metzger McQuiston
Private Practice

Adele A. Webb
College of Nursing, University of Akron

The purpose of this series of monographs is to provide the reader with a concise description of conceptual frameworks and theories in nursing. It is not intended to replace the primary works of nurse theorists, but to provide direction for their use. Designed for undergraduate students, these monographs will also be helpful guides for graduate students and faculty.

Due to the complexity of existing books and chapters on nursing conceptual frameworks and theories, students often have difficulty understanding and incorporating nursing theory into their practice. The concise monographs of this series include a biographical sketch of the theorist, origin of the theory, assumptions, concepts, propositions, examples for application to practice and research, glossary of terms, and a bibliography of classic works, critiques, and research. Organization of the information in this manner will facilitate student understanding and use, thereby broadening the base of nursing science.

ROSEMARIE PARSE

Theory of Health as Human Becoming

Sheila Bunting

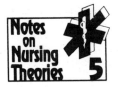

Notes
on
Nursing
Theories 5

SAGE Publications
International Educational and Professional Publisher
Newbury Park   London   New Delhi

For information address:

SAGE Publications, Inc.
2455 Teller Road
Newbury Park, California 91320

SAGE Publications Ltd.
6 Bonhill Street
London EC2A 4PU
United Kingdom

SAGE Publications India Pvt. Ltd.
M-32 Market
Greater Kailash I
New Delhi 110 048 India

Printed in the United States of America

Library of Congress Cataloging-in-Publication Data

Bunting, Sheila.
  Rosemarie Parse: theory of health as human becoming / Sheila Bunting.
    p.   cm.—(Notes on nursing theories; v. 5)
  Includes bibliographical references.
  ISBN 0-8039-4795-X (cl.).—ISBN 0-8039-4549-3 (pbk.)
  1. Nursing—Philosophy. 2. Parse, Rosemarie Rizzo. I. Title.
II. Series.
  [DNLM: 1. Parse, Rosemarie Rizzo. 2. Nursing Care. 3. Nursing Theory. 4. Philosophy, Nursing. WY 86 B942r]
  RT84.5.B85   1993
  610.73—dc20
  DNLM/DLC   92-49481
                                                                  CIP

93 94 95 96 10 9 8 7 6 5 4 3 2 1

Sage Production Editor: Megan M. McCue

This monograph is lovingly and gratefully dedicated
to my mother, Pauline Wilson McGuire,
a person who has always been open to the possibles
and has participated with me in my becoming.

Contents

Foreword

There are those nursing leaders among us who call us to question
our traditions and stretch our boundaries beyond what *is* to what
is possible for nursing's contribution to the health of humankind.
Rosemarie Parse is one such leader. In her theory of human becoming she presents a conceptualization of nursing as a professional
discipline—a basic science—focusing on the study of the human
health experience. This science assigns nursing practice the goal of
enhancing the quality of life as defined by our clients. Our clients
become the experts on their health and their lives. They are not
passive recipients of our care but instead are involved creators of
their health. From this perspective, health cannot be assessed or
diagnosed by the nurse. Health is a way of living according to
personal values that reflects the unique process of becoming. Nursing practice, according to Parse, is being in relationship, in true
loving presence, with clients while they describe the meaning of
their lifeworld, struggle with the paradoxes inherent in health
experiences, and discover and fulfill hopes and dreams.

This monograph provides an overview of Parse's foundational
beliefs and theoretical constructs. Sheila Bunting may be congrat-
ulated for her summary and provocative presentation that continually invite students to explore the primary sources of the cited
theory texts, practice examples, and research for deeper under-
standings. This work may be used as a springboard for study of

the theory of human becoming. It introduces beginning students to the philosophical underpinnings, the assumptions about the nature of persons and health, the specific conceptual and propositional formulations of the theory, and the applications in practice and research. In addition, Parse's particular practice and research methodologies are briefly described. Through her examples, Bunting seeks to lead students beyond the language and structure of the theory toward a grasp of its profound message and the uniqueness of the nursing practice that it generates.

Theories are not static entities "cast in stone," or in this case, "cast in print," in their original versions. Theories are dynamic; they change and grow as they are nurtured by the scholars who work with them in practice and in research. Since the original publication of *Man-Living-Health: A Theory of Nursing* in 1981, Parse has continued to modify and further develop the theory of human becoming. The theory has been adopted as a framework for practice by nurses throughout the world. Several evaluation studies have documented differences in client perceptions of quality of life, nurses' perceptions of their practice, and administrators' perceptions of morale and the quality of nursing practice following a 6- to 9-month implementation of Parse's theory in practice. The theory has been used as the philosophical and theoretical perspective of many master's theses and doctoral dissertations. Published research continues to contribute to the growth of the theory.

This monograph is a "snapshot" of Parse's theory in 1992. It is a glimpse into a distinctive world of nursing framed with respect for the mystery of health and the wonder of human becoming.

MARLAINE C. SMITH, RN, PHD
University of Colorado
School of Nursing

Acknowledgments

I would like to thank Dr. Marlaine Smith for her support and encouragement and for her patience and care in the reading and rereading of this manuscript. Dr. Louette Lutjens and editor Dr. Adele Webb, old friends and classmates, served as guides, offering long distance counseling and advice at odd hours. I am grateful to Dr. Rosemarie Rizzo Parse for her past mentorship, for the assistance she has extended to me in my pursuit of this project, and, most particularly, for her theory, so grandly conceptualized and beautifully written, and for its potential to empower clients and enrich nursing.

Biographical Sketch of the Nurse Theorist: Rosemarie Rizzo Parse, PhD, RN, FAAN

Position: Professor and Coordinator of the Center for Nursing
    Research, Hunter College, New York
President of Discovery International, Inc.
Editor: *Nursing Science Quarterly*
BSN: Duquesne University, Pittsburgh
MS: University of Pittsburgh
PhD: University of Pittsburgh
Fellow: American Academy of Nursing

SOURCE: (Lee & Schumacher, 1989)

1

Origins of the Theory

Historical Evolution of the Theory

Parse has pointed out that the discipline of nursing has traditionally been grounded in the natural sciences such as chemistry,
physics, and physiology, and that it has been guided by the medical model in its practice. She proposed the theory of human becoming (formerly called Man-Living-Health) as an alternative framework. This theory synthesized concepts from Rogers's conceptual
system and major ideas from the existential-phenomenological
philosophies of Heidegger, Sartre, Merleau-Ponty, and Marcel
(Parse, 1981, p. 5).

Heidegger was a German philosopher who died in 1976. He was
interested in analyzing the complexity of human existence, which
he termed *Dasein*, meaning "being there" (Heidegger, 1962). The
term *Dasein* signifies both the mystery and the randomness or
chance associated with being in the world in a given time and
place. Despite this view of the arbitrary nature of human existence,
Heidegger focused on the freedom he believed each person pos-
sessed. This freedom included the choice to live authentically and
to recognize the limits of one's human nature and confront the fact
of one's nonbeing. This acceptance of one's finite existence and
one's own death makes possible a life of conscience, care, and
responsibility. Living authentically is discovering oneself in direct

relation to the existing world. To live authentically, one must make the choice to do so, to reject the world of tasks, rules, and the urgency of external standards. "In choosing to make this choice, Dasein *makes possible* . . . its authentic potentiality-for-Being" (Heidegger, 1962, p. 313). An important part of existential-phenomenological philosophy is the view of time. The authentic present involves the dynamic interplay of the past and future; it is related to a past that one is reliving in the present, and a future anticipated as a present reality. The concepts of freedom, authenticity, and this multidimensional quality of time are important in Parse's theory. Other writers whose works presented the existential-phenomenological movement to the public included Jean-Paul Sartre (1956) and Maurice Merleau-Ponty (1962).

Parse believed that the medical model view of the person was that of a mechanistic being, and that medicine traditionally treated the person in a fragmented manner. The particulate or *sum of parts* view is a logical extension of the view of the person as a collection of separate parts, called *Cartesian psychophysical dualism* (Lavine, 1984) after Rene Descartes. Descartes was a philosopher who believed in two separate kinds of reality. One was a physical substance that had no consciousness and took up space, and the other was a thinking, spiritual substance that, by definition, had no physical extension. In this view, the mind and spirit can be separated from the body.

The offering of an alternative to this *sum of parts* view of the person that had been maintained by many areas of medicine and nursing required a major change of perspective. Such a shift occurred when the work of Martha Rogers provided a unitary perspective of the human being and a new way to see the role of nursing (Rogers, 1970). Parse's theory is partially derived from this nursing framework.

Parse's ideas were influenced by her own nursing experiences involving teaching and persuading patients to do things that medical experts deemed "good for them." She concluded that the patients had their own reality and behaved accordingly (Parse, 1985a). The early premises of her theory appeared in her first book, *Nursing Fundamentals* (Parse, 1974). These premises included statements related to the focus and methods that should be the concern of nurses, the nature of the human being, and the important construct of the mutual, interactive manner in which the human and the environment evolve together (Parse, 1974; Smith & Hudepohl, 1988). During the early development of her theory in the 1970s, Parse was a member of the faculty at Duquesne University where there was an internationally recognized center in existential phenomenology. The study of and interactions with these philosophers formed a basis for the synthesis of the elements of these concepts within the assumptions of her theory (R. R. Parse, personal communication, April 1987; Smith & Hudepohl, 1988). The purpose of Parse's theory was to create a paradigm (or model guideline) of nursing rooted in the human sciences. She saw the human sciences as being directed toward uncovering the meaning of events in the lives of persons as these events were experienced by the persons themselves—the study of the human being's participative experience in a situation. In creating this theory, she synthesized Rogers's principles of helicy, complementarity (now called integrality), and resonancy, and the building blocks of energy field, openness, pattern and organization, and four-dimensionality with the tenets and concepts of existential phenomenology (Parse, 1981, p. 13).

Martha Rogers's principle of integrality describes human beings and their environments as integrated and interacting energy fields that are continuously and mutually changing. These human and environmental fields are identified, according to Rogers's theory, by patterns and organizations of wave frequencies that are continuously changing "from lower-frequency, longer wave patterns to higher-frequency, shorter wave patterns" (Rogers, 1980, p. 333). Rogers termed this concept of changing waves and patterns *resonancy*. The direction of that change—Rogers's principle of *helicy*—is always new and always moving toward greater complexity, never going backwards or repeating its pattern. Rogers was very clear in specifying the open nature of the human and environmental fields. "Man and environment are continually exchanging matter and energy with one another" (Rogers, 1970, p. 54).

Parse's theory, then, has its base in Rogers's Science of Unitary Human Beings. Rogers's conceptual system, in turn, is rooted in humanistic as well as natural scientific thought. The basic statements of Parse's theory were written at a philosophical level from a combination of existential-phenomenological ideas (the tenets of subjectivity and intentionality and the concepts of coconstitution, coexistence, and situated freedom) synthesized with Rogers's principles and building blocks (Parse, 1987, p. 161).

The tenet of human *subjectivity* refers to the person as a conscious being who is capable of encountering the world, relating to it, and growing from the relationship. The human can and does give meaning to all of the things that occur between him or herself and the world, thereby taking an active part in creating and constituting the reality of both the self and the world. The tenet of *intentionality* means that the person is knowingly open to the world. To be human is to be intentionally involved with and present to the world (Parse, 1981). *Situated freedom* refers to the belief that one chooses the situations in which one finds oneself as well as one's attitude and response to the situations. The way in which a particular situation comes about and develops is related to the previous choices of that individual. The tenet of free choice for human beings has been synthesized by Parse from the work of Sartre (1956) and is an important element of her theory. *Coexistence* means that life as a person knows it is an experience of being with others. One is brought into the world by other beings and one's perceptions of self and the environment are formed with the input of others. "Without others one would not know that one is" or who one is (Parse, 1981, p. 20). *Coconstitution* signifies that the reality of any situation is related to all of the elements that make up that situation and the meaning assigned by the person. To say that humans coconstitute situations is to say that their perceptions, together with the other elements of the situation, create the reality. By being present in a situation and being in relationship to the multiple views of the world and others in the world, the individual influences these views and takes part in the *cocreation* of the situation and of the world.

The evolution of Parse's theory, synthesized from the elements of Rogers's framework and those of existential-phenomenology, is illustrated in Figure 1.1.

Important differences between Rogers's and Parse's conceptualizations are the differing views of the human being and of health. Parse viewed the person as an open being who cocreates personal health rather than viewing the person as an energy field. She viewed health as a "process of becoming as experienced and described by the person" whereas Rogers viewed health as a value (Parse, 1992, p. 36). The human capacity to participate and shape the environment, to freely choose meaning in a situation, to take responsibility for choices and decisions, to mutually shape patterns of relating and existing,

Rogers		Existential Phenomenology	
Principles	Concepts	Concepts	Tenets
Helicy Complimentarity Resonancy	Energy Field Openness Pattern and Organization	Coconstitution Coexistence Situated Freedom	Intentionality Human Subjectivity

Assumptions

Human	Becoming
1. The human is coexisting while coconstituting rhythmical patterns with the universe.	5. Becoming is an open process experienced by the human.
2. The human is an open being, freely choosing meaning in situation, bearing responsibility for decisions.	6. Becoming is a rhythmically coconstituting process of human-universe interrelationship.
3. The human is a living unity continuously coconstituting patterns of relating.	7. Becoming is the human's pattern of relating value priorities.
4. The human is transcending multidimensionally with the possibles.	8. Becoming is an intersubjective process of transcending with the possibles.
	9. Becoming is human unfolding.

Principles

1. Structuring meaning multidimensionally is cocreating reality through the languaging of valuing and imaging.	2. Cocreating rhythmical patterns of relating is living the paradoxical unity of revealing-concealing and enabling-limiting while connecting-separating.	3. Cotranscending with the possibles is powering unique ways of originating in the process of transforming.

Figure 1.1. Evolution of the Theory of Human Becoming
SOURCE: Adapted from Parse (1992).

and to transcend beyond the present reality is central to Parse's theory and to her conceptualization of the person.

Dr. Parse continues to develop her theory through her own research and by working closely with other nursing scholars. This includes the mentoring of students, many of whom have used her theory to guide their theses and doctoral dissertations (see listings in the bibliography). The primary texts of her work are *Man-Living-Health: A Theory of Nursing* (Parse, 1981) and the chapter, "Man-Living-Health Theory of Nursing" in Parse's edited book, *Nursing Science: Major Paradigms, Theories and Critiques* (Parse, 1987). An excellent precis and update on the language of her theory appeared in a recent article in *Nursing Science Quarterly* (Parse, 1992).

2

Assumptions

Described in Parse's 1981 book and presented with updated language in 1992, the central conceptual units from Rogers's framework along with those from existential phenomenology are synthesized into nine assumptions (Parse, 1992, p. 38). (See Figure 1.1.) These assumptions state beliefs about human beings and health; five address human beings and four address health as human becoming.

Assumptions of a theory are statements that are accepted or assumed to be true without requiring proof. They are statements of foundational beliefs on which the theory is built. In selecting a theory to guide practice or research, an individual must first be sure that the assumptions of the theory are in agreement with his or her worldview. For instance, if one believes in absolute cause and effect, Parse's assumptions would not fit with one's worldview. Parse's theory is based on a belief that events and people mutually shape and influence one another. The idea of health as the person adapting to or coping with the environment is inconsistent with Parse's theory (Parse, 1987). In the theory of human becoming, the view that a person has a part in creating his or her own reality affects both the accepted assumptions and the basic principles of the theory. Parse stated that the most significant distinction of her theory from that of other nursing theorists is the belief that the human being, who is more than and different from the sum of the parts, "evolves mutually with the environment, participates in cocreating personal health by choosing meanings in situations, and conveys meanings that are personal values reflecting dreams and hopes" (Parse, 1987, p. 162).

In discussing the language used in her theory, originally called Man-Living-Health, Parse stated that the word *man* referred to *homo sapiens*, or the human being in general, rather than to males only. She frequently uses participles and gerunds (verbs ending in "ing") to call attention to the fact that her theory deals with things that are in process (Parse, 1987), that is, they are happening as one thinks about them.

Assumption 1. "The human is coexisting while coconstituting rhythmical patterns with the universe" (Parse, 1992, p. 38). The meaning of the first assumption is that the individual exists with other persons, evolving as the universe is evolving. The patterns formed by the person exchanging energy with the universe are unique to that person. These particular patterns of relating distinguish an individual from the environmental pattern and from the patterns of all other persons in the universe. The person, then, "is a pattern of patterns of relating . . . the individual's unique way of being recognized" (Parse, 1981, p. 26). Important in Parse's theory is the active part taken by individuals in creating their own patterns and their own reality.

Assumption 2. "The human is an open being, freely choosing meaning in situation, bearing responsibility for decisions" (Parse, 1992, p. 38). This statement signifies that the human being *chooses* ways of being in a situation and is accountable for those choices. By choosing some meanings of the situations of his or her life and not choosing others, the individual opens many possibilities and closes others. These losses and gains, the "birthings and dyings . . . are the rhythmical happenings in day-to-day living" (Parse, 1981, p. 27). The events of a person's life and the meanings of those events are created as the individual, through the choices made, creates the possibilities that he or she can become. Even when people do not know the outcomes of the choices they make, they are responsible for those outcomes. Persons and the universe exchange energy to make the world. The individual chooses the meaning given to the situations he or she cocreates.

Assumption 3. "The human is a living unity continuously co-constituting patterns of relating" (Parse, 1992, p. 38). The idea of the human as a living unity means that he or she is more than and different from the sum of the parts, that is the physiological, psychological, spiritual, sociological, and other classifications that are often assigned to dimensions of the person. Coconstitution is the individual's "active participation in creating meaning with others in the world" (Parse, 1981, p. 177). This meaning is created in the interactions that occur between individuals and their world. These coconstituted patterns of relating are the unitary person's ways of being. The patterns are expressed and identified "through gesture, movement, gaze, posture, touch, and speech" (Parse, 1981, p. 28). One can distinguish a person from all others in the universe by the patterns of appearance, mannerisms, voice, and other characteristics that make the person individual.

Assumption 4. "The human is transcending multidimensionally with the possibles" (Parse, 1992, p. 38). *Transcending* means "going beyond, exceeding" (Parse, 1981, p. 179). *Multidimensionality* "refers to human existence as beyond the temporo-spatial limits of a three-dimensional universe" (Marlaine Smith, personal communication, October 1991). There are many levels of the universe experienced by a person simultaneously. Specifically, Parse (1987) refers to this concept as "explicit-tacit knowing" (p. 162). She pointed out that not all choices are made from the explicit level and that humans construct their meanings from a "whole sense of the situation" (Parse, 1987, p. 162). Cognitive logic and thought, along with the intuitive "hunch", are experienced by the person as a unified impression all at once. The human being is capable of moving beyond the present reality, of growing and becoming something more and different from what the present limits may indicate. The choices to grow to new possible dimensions are decided from many types of knowledge, including a logical deductive reflection and a "prereflective" grasp of the situation.

Assumption 5. "Becoming is an open process, experienced by the human" (Parse, 1992, p. 38). The process of becoming is the human being's continuous growing through exchange of energy with the universe, and this process of becoming is health in Parse's theory. This process of health involves continuous change. The direction of change evolves toward more diversity and more complexity. As persons grow and develop they become more different from one another, more complicated and more intricate. Part of the process of growing is choosing who one will be in a given situation (Parse, 1981). These choices are unique and personal and they determine reality for a person: "An experience of a situation, while cocreated with others, belongs to one human being only" (Parse, 1981, p. 30). The person creates health by the choices made. Choosing some options automatically eliminates other options, so the person cocreates and experiences possibilities within a different perspective as he or she participates in the process of becoming, living health (Parse, 1981). Each time one makes a choice there are many things that are not chosen, some that one knows about and many that one does not or cannot know. Health, then, is cocreated by a person's choices.

Assumption 6. "Becoming is a rhythmically coconstituting process of the human-universe interrelationship" (Parse, 1992, p. 38). This assumption means that health, the process of becoming, is a continuous energy interchange created both by the human and the universe (cocreated) as they interrelate (Parse, 1981, pp. 30-31). Change occurs in this becoming and change involves an ongoing process of connecting with some things while separating from others. The human's health "is the rhythmic process of changing through the simultaneous connecting and separating" (Parse, 1987, p. 31) of the person with the environment. The people, beliefs, events, and other elements of the environment, which we connect with and separate from, change us and are changed by us in an ongoing rhythm. With all of these elements we coconstitute our health.

Assumption 7. "Becoming is the human's pattern of relating value priorities" (Parse, 1992, p. 38). This assumption means that health (human becoming) is the individual's way of living the particular ideals chosen and cherished by that person. Health is a synthesis of the values of an individual (Parse, 1987, p. 31). The choices the individual makes are an expression of cherished values and ways of relating and being. "These ways of being emerge in recognizable patterns" (Parse, 1981, p. 32). The way of being brings out emerging patterns that indicate the priorities and increasing complexity of each human being. These emerging patterns make up the individual's health.

Assumption 8. "Becoming is an intersubjective process of transcending with the possibles" (Parse, 1992, p. 38). This assumption, a statement about health as human becoming, "means that health is reaching beyond the actual to the possible through subject-to-subject energy interchange" (Parse, 1981, p. 32). Though *intersubjective* means between two separate conscious minds, in this assumption this interchange can and does occur between humans and other elements in the universe as well as between human beings. The genuine relating to another person is a risk, and it reflects individuals choosing ways of becoming more complex and more diverse. It means giving up the familiar to "struggle with the unfamiliar toward an imaged not-yet" (Parse, 1981, p. 32) as individuals reveal and conceal who they are and who they can become.

Assumption 9. "Becoming is human unfolding" (Parse, 1992, p. 38). This assumption means that health is the process of the human being "synergistically becoming more complex and more diverse in coexistence with others" (Parse, 1981, p. 33). Human becoming as an unfolding involves open systems exchanging energy and changing continuously, never going backwards or returning to a previous state. This idea of health proposes that health is "a non-specific entity, continuously transforming" (Parse, 1981, p. 33) as the human being grows older. An important element in Parse's definition of health is that it is an ongoing process of the individual being with others. All humans and other elements of the universe are unfolding toward greater complexity.

Parse, in her 1987 book, further synthesized her nine assumptions into three assumptions. These are listed and discussed below.
1. Human becoming "is freely choosing personal meaning in situations in the intersubjective process of relating value priorities" (Parse, 1987, p. 161). In explaining this assumption, Parse stated that the human being, "through subject-to-subject-interchange in situation assigns meaning which reflects personal values" (Parse, 1987, p. 161). Because more than one meaning can always be given to any event or action, the meaning that one chooses to give is determined by the individual's values and previous experiences. The

person does not, however, assign these meanings in isolation. Meanings are always affected by communication with others in a person's life; that is, the meanings are created intersubjectively. An example of different meanings given to an event might be those assigned by persons taking a morning walk. To person A it is a chore she is forcing herself to do, to person B it is a gift of time for herself to be alone before she starts the day, and to person C it is the means of getting to a meeting with her lover. Because Parse's definition of health is that of a process, a personal choosing of meaning which cocreates reality with the universe, each of these persons can be seen as expressing cherished values and ways of relating and being. These emerging patterns make up the individual's health.

2. Human becoming "is cocreating rhythmical patterns of relating in open interchange with the environment" (Parse, 1987, p. 162). This means the person-universe interrelationship is reflected in the patterns created together. One can distinguish and recognize the human and the environment by their patterns. Parse stated that the human, together with universe, creates the pattern of each. The human is distinguishable as human and environment as environment, "yet each is a coparticipant in the creation of the other" (Parse, 1987, p. 162). An example of this concept is a woman who lives in an intermediate care residence for the elderly. As she interrelates in her new setting, both she and the community of residents and attendants are mutually changing. Together they evolve patterns of being alone and together.

3. Human becoming "is cotranscending multidimensionally with the unfolding possibles" (Parse, 1987, p. 162). This means that human becoming is "moving beyond self at all levels of the universe as dreams become actualities" (Parse, 1987, p. 162). *Cotranscending* means "going beyond the actual in interrelationship with others" (Parse, 1987, p. 166). *Multidimensionally* refers to the various levels of the universe that are experienced simultaneously (Parse, 1987, p. 162). Or, it is all the ways that a person can "know" as a unified impression. An example might be a family working with a child with special health needs. As the family members work with the child and with one another, each moves beyond the self and the present reality to the possibles that unfold. This movement beyond is not a linear development but occurs on many levels at once (multidimensionally). The family's health is the movement toward and the expression of these possibles as they are chosen and lived.

3

Concepts, Principles, and Theoretical Structures

According to Parse, the major themes emerging from the philosophical assumptions are meaning, rhythmicity, and cotranscendence (moving beyond with another). Each theme leads to the development of a principle of human becoming. The understanding of concepts unique to Parse's work is essential to comprehension of her theory.

Major Concepts

The principles of Parse's theory of human becoming contain nine major concepts, three from each of the principles. They are imaging, valuing, languaging, revealing-concealing, enabling-limiting, connecting-separating, powering, originating, and transforming. These are all processes in which individuals actively engage.

"What is real for each individual is structured by that individual" (Parse, 1992, p. 37). *Imaging* refers to knowing in the many ways a person can know something. It is the creating of perceptions (internal pictures, feelings, sounds) of events, ideas, and people—making them real. This creation of reality includes one's images of the past and the future as well as constructions of the present. In *languaging*, one communicates perceptions, beliefs, and priorities through verbal and nonverbal means—"Sharing valued images through symbols of words, gesture, gaze, touch, and posture" (Parse, 1981, p. 177). *Valuing* is "the process of living cherished beliefs while assimilating the new into a personal worldview. It emerges in the human-universe process and is the human being's confirming of cherished beliefs" (Parse, 1992, p. 37). By the life that one lives and the choices one makes, one expresses and testifies to one's beliefs and values.

Parse's paradoxical concepts concern the merging of seeming opposites in which the dialectical processes are occurring simultaneously. These processes can be thought of as background/foreground concepts. That is, one cannot think of one without implicitly summoning up the idea of the other, as the idea of noise is present in silence, and the idea of white in thinking of the color black. *Connecting-separating*, according to Parse, "is the rhythmical process of distancing and relating, that is, moving in one direction and away from others, yet always toward greater diversity" (Parse, 1987, p. 164). Each choice made brings a person closer to certain elements of the universe and farther from others. One meets different people and lives different experiences each year (or day) of one's life. This year is lived differently than last year, but the past experiences are now part of the living person, and he or she therefore has become more diverse and will continue to become more diverse. Connecting with some events and people and separating from others creates a rhythmic pattern because all connections and separations are related.

Connecting-separating with people and projects is *enabling-limiting* (Parse, 1987, p. 164) because each connection or separation choice contains a number of possibilities and also many limitations. Each road taken represents many roads one was unable to take. Each change that one makes in life enables one to envision new possibilities and limits one in the pursuit of other possibilities. As one relates to others, one is always *revealing-concealing* the personal self. One can never completely reveal the whole of the self to another, so the concealing is always there as a part of the revealing process. By choosing to reveal, one selects at the same time what one will conceal.

Parse's concept of *powering* is the energizing force behind creativity, the drive that provides the fuel to allow change and creativity to happen. "Powering is the pushing-resisting of interhuman encounters" (Parse, 1987, p. 165). *Originating* is creating and generating new and different ways of being in the world. Persons are originating when they initiate new patterns of interrelationships with their universes. Parse (1987) defines *transforming* as "the changing of change"(p. 165). Change itself is a continuous process of the human-universe interrelationship. It can be recognized by its ever increasing variety. The transcending, or moving beyond, which occurs through transforming, takes place through struggling. Transforming, or changing, "unfolds as the familiar is seen in a different light, thus shifting the view and illuminating new possibles" (Parse, 1987, p. 165).

Principles

Principle 1. "Structuring meaning multidimensionally is cocreating reality through the languaging of valuing and imaging" (Parse, 1987, p. 163). Principle 1 connects and relates Parse's concepts of imaging, valuing, and languaging. Structuring meaning multidimensionally signifies that individuals construct their meaning of situations from many levels of the universe, from an "explicit-tacit knowing" (Parse, 1987, p. 162). Not all choices are made from the explicit level; humans construct their meanings from a "whole sense of the situation" (Parse, 1987, p. 162; see Assumption 4). Individuals, by the choices they make between meanings, are active in cocreating (with their universe and the people around them) their personal reality. "Health is an expression of values at the moment, the meaning given to a situation" (Parse, 1987, p. 163).

Illustration: A young man who was recently diagnosed with AIDS feels devastated and helpless. He is confronting, on many levels, the meanings he has created from all that he knows from others' comments, what he has read, and from his own sense of the situation (structuring meaning multidimensionally). While talking to the nurse about his past life, his present, and his hopes for the future (languaging), he begins to see different meanings (cocreated reality). He is able to envision the past and present of his life and the different meanings he has constructed (imaging), realizing that he has been able and is presently able to live his cherished beliefs (valuing).

Principle 2. "Cocreating rhythmical patterns of relating is living the paradoxical unity of revealing-concealing, enabling-limiting, while connecting-separating" (Parse, 1987, p. 164). The human and the universe, including the people in one's life, cocreate a rhythmical interchange. As each person grows and changes, she or he forms bonds with some aspects of the universe, including people, places, and activities, and simultaneously breaks bonds with others. Other persons and elements in the universe are moving toward and away from one another as well, revealing aspects of themselves while concealing other aspects in an ongoing rhythmical pattern of interrelationships. Each pattern of the kaleidoscope is different, more complex, containing elements of all of the previous patterns.

Illustration: In order to be close by for her mother, whose dementia was becoming a safety factor, a woman made the decision to leave her valued and stimulating position in an office to do her work on consignment out of her home. She was conscious of separating from her former valued associates while connecting with new contacts and connecting in a new way with personal friends and family, particularly her daughters, who offered to help care for their grandmother. Her new work situation was enabling in that her time schedule was more open, but it was more limiting in its constrictions on her movements outside her home. She found herself relating differently to persons who had always known her as a person who worked outside the home. In her rhythmical interchanges with the persons who questioned her about her situation, she was aware of revealing some of the new meanings she had created while concealing others.

Principle 3. "Cotranscending with the possibles is powering unique ways of originating in the process of transforming" (Parse, 1987, p. 165). Parse's concepts of powering (energizing), originating (creating anew), and transforming (changing change) are related in this principle. Cotranscending is "going beyond the actual in interrelationship with others" (Parse, 1987, p. 166). The presence of others may help persons to move beyond the perceived limits of the present, though the person must do the moving herself or himself. This is an important concept because nurses can help clients move beyond. The actual impetus, or energy, for the moving beyond is termed *powering* by Parse. Moving beyond the present reality with other persons is energizing the creation of new realities in the process of making changes.

Illustration: A couple in a relationship involving spouse abuse expressed the desire to change their abusive pattern and to move beyond it together. The husband, a trainee in a very demanding executive development program for his new job, tended to cease interacting with his wife when he was panicked about his work. The wife valued intimacy and had a pattern of open communication of feelings. Faced with an unresponsive husband, her own anxiety led her to push him to talk about his feelings and resist his request to be left alone. He abused her verbally and struck her in the face.

Both parties valued the relationship and wanted to develop new ways of living together. They began to question the meanings of the connections and familiar patterns of their relating. As they talked about these meanings, they found themselves struggling with their past images and their expectations of one another in the present and future. The meanings began to transform, moving beyond the familiar to a new image of how they could be together.

Theoretical Structures

Parse's definition of a theoretical structure is "a statement interrelating concepts in a way that can be verified" (Parse, 1981, p. 68). Theoretical structures are "nondirectional propositions," which are "noncausal in nature and consistent with the assumptions and principles [of Parse's theory]" (Parse, 1987, p. 166). They are designed to guide practice and research. To make these operational in practice and research, "statements about nursing practice must be derived and lived experiences chosen for study" (Parse, 1987, p. 166). Parse suggested that it is appropriate to use one concept from each principle to derive a theoretical structure. The relationships between concepts, principles, and the three theoretical structures that have been derived and published are illustrated in Figure 3.1.

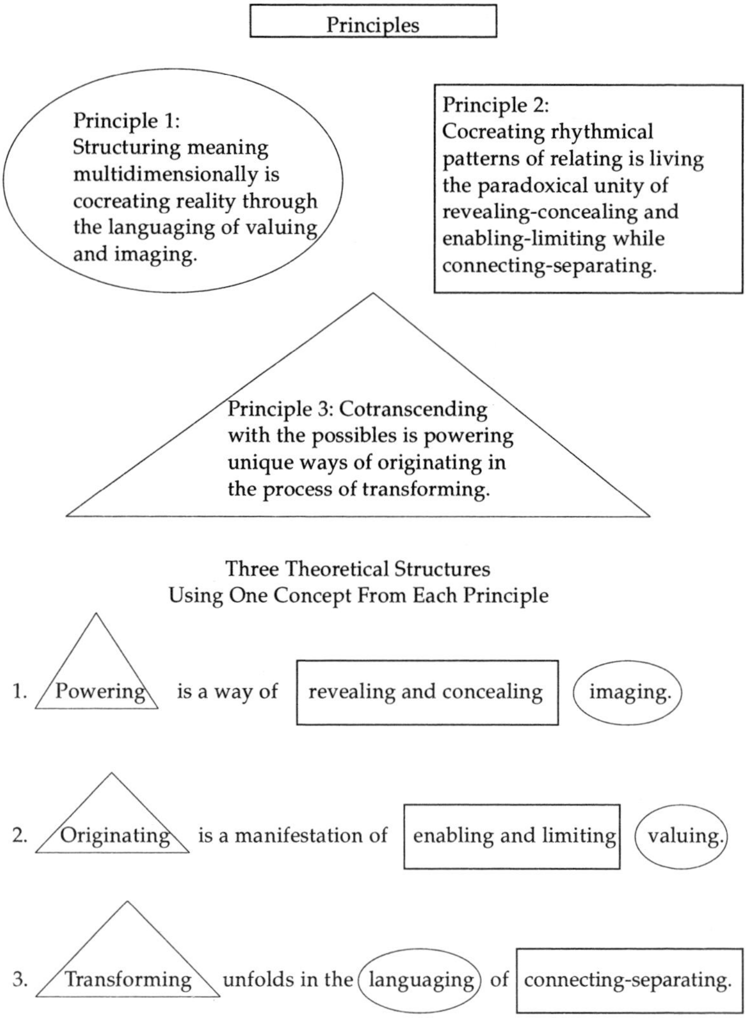

Figure 3.1. Derivation of Theoretical Structures From Principles and Concepts of the Theory of Human Becoming
SOURCE: Adapted from Parse (1992).

4

Major Nursing Concepts

The Simultaneity Paradigm

Four major concepts of concern to nursing are (a) the persons or groups who benefit from nursing services, (b) their environment, (c) their health, and (d) nursing. To describe the ways in which these concepts are viewed in Rogers's and Parse's nursing theories, Parse created the term *simultaneity paradigm*, which indicates different ways of looking at the human being, health, and the goals of nursing (Parse, 1987, pp. 136-137). The word *paradigm* indicates a way of thinking about concepts and their relationships, "a way of viewing a particular field of study" (Parse, 1981, p. 178). The condition of *simultaneity* is, according to the dictionary, the happening of two or more events at the same time. The term emphasizes that the concepts in Parse's theory are ever in process, always becoming. The naming of the simultaneity paradigm came from the consideration of the human being within this paradigm as "a synergistic being in open, mutual, simultaneous interchange with the environment" (Parse, 1985b, p. 1).

The person, as viewed in the simultaneity paradigm, is thought of as different from and more than the sum of parts. He or she is able to take part knowingly in the process of change, interacting continuously with the universe in a mutual, integral exchange of matter and energy. Health is seen as a process experienced by the person and unique to that person, not as a condition, a state, or an outcome. The goal of nursing in the simultaneity paradigm is service to persons (Rogers, 1987), focusing on the quality of life as the individual perceives it, regardless of society's designation of illness (Parse, 1987, pp. 136-137).

Human Becoming

Parse's man-living-health nursing theory has been renamed the *human becoming theory*. No changes have been made in the theory itself. The change in name reflects the change in the dictionary definition of *man*, which is now the male human (Parse, 1992). In 1980, when *Man-Living-Health: A Theory of Nursing* was being written, *man* was defined as the generic human. The putting together of *man, living,* and *health* into a hyphenated whole "creates a unity of meaning different from the individual words as they stand alone" (Parse, 1981, p. 39). The combined words make it clear that human health is the ongoing process of participation with the world. Man-Living-Health is a unitary phenomenon that refers to the person's becoming through cocreating rhythmical patterns of relating as energy is exchanged with the environment. Health, then, is a process of the human being relating to his or her universe, and it is created by the person and the universe together. Health in this theory is not thought of separately from the person and the environment.

> Health is Man's unfolding. It is Man's lived experiences, a nonlinear entity that cannot be qualified by terms such as good, bad, more, or less. It is not Man adapting or coping. Unitary Man's health is a synthesis of values, a way of living. It is not the opposite of disease or a state that man has, but rather is a continuously changing process that Man cocreates. (Parse, 1987, p. 160)

Nursing

Nursing as a process would not be included within the theoretical metaparadigm concepts in Parse's theory. *Nursing* is defined in Parse's theory as "a discipline focusing on the study of the

Dimensions	Processes
1. Illuminating meaning is shedding light through uncovering the what was, is, and will be, as it is appearing now. It happens in explicating what is.	1. Explicating is making clear what is appearing now through languaging.
2. Synchronizing rhythms happens in dwelling with the pitch, yaw, and roll of the interhuman cadence.	2. Dwelling with is giving self over to the flow of the struggle in connecting-separating.
3. Mobilizing transcendence happens in moving beyond the meaning moment to what is not yet.	3. Moving beyond is propelling toward the possibles in transforming.

Figure 4.1. The Theory of Human Becoming Practice Methodology
SOURCE: Adapted from Parse (1992).

health of persons in interrelationship with their environment" (Marlaine C. Smith, personal communication, October 1991). Nursing practice was described by Parse as involving both science and art: "It is the utilization of nursing's abstract body of knowledge in the service to people" (Parse, 1981, p. 81). The reponsibility of nursing to society is to guide the choosing of possibilities in the changing health process. This guiding occurs through an intersubjective participation with persons and their families. The goal of nursing is to enhance the quality of life as perceived by the person and the family (Parse, 1987, p. 167).

Parse rejected the nursing process as not evolving from the science of nursing (Parse, 1987, p. 166). Dimensions of practice are illuminating meaning, synchronizing rhythms, and mobilizing transcendence. The processes Parse advocated for nursing practice are (a) explicating, defined as making clear what is appearing now through languaging; (b) dwelling with, which is giving self over to the flow of the struggle in connecting-separating; and (c) moving beyond, which is propelling toward the possibles in transforming (Parse, 1987, p. 169). The dimensions and processes of nurses practicing within the theory of human becoming are listed in Figure 4.1.

Parse stated that the person is an open being who freely chooses "meaning in situation and bears responsibility for the choices"

(Parse, 1981, p. 39). Parse was very clear that the values of the individual must predominate and that the nurse serves in a supportive role rather than serving as the authority figure who knows and tells what is best for the person. Individuals are the experts on themselves and their health, and they are responsible and autonomous. Their judgments and their views are the significant ones.

5

Practice Methodologies

The methodology recommended for the theory of human becoming is a selection of dimensions and processes that are different from the nursing process (Mitchell & Santopinto, 1988). The practice methodology of human becoming is unlike the nursing process in which nurses, in assessing, ask specific questions of their clients and identify problems associated with isolated causal agents. The nurses then plan, carry out, and evaluate interventions. In nursing practice guided by the theory of human becoming, nurses do not "diagnose" or fit clients into preestablished categories, nor do they label any phenomena as "problems." There are no assumptions of linear cause and effect. The dimensions of the practice methodology for the theory of human becoming are related to Parse's three principles.

Illuminating Meaning

Principle 1, which is structuring meaning multidimensionally, gives rise to the dimension "Illuminating meaning through explicating" (Parse, 1987, p. 168). "Illuminating meaning involves shedding light through the uncovering" (Parse, 1987, p. 168) of the meaning of the past, the present, and the future from the client's/family's perspective. As clients talk about their meanings, the communicating of the impressions, thoughts, and feelings changes

25

the meanings, making them more clear and explicit. This is accomplished by *languaging*, which is the sharing of their ideas and perceptions through words, gestures, facial expressions, touch, and body language (Parse, 1981, p. 177). The process related to this dimension is the nursing activity of explicating, which is "making clear what is appearing now through languaging" (Parse, 1987, p. 167). Thinking about and expressing to the nurse the thoughts and feelings connected with this moment in time can lead the client/family to a new way of viewing the familiar situation, allowing them to use new aspects of the universe in cocreating a different ongoing reality.

Synchronizing Rhythms

The dimension of "synchronizing rhythms through dwelling with the ebb and flow of human encounters" (Parse, 1987, p. 167) comes from Principle 2—cocreating rhythmical patterns. Parse observed that there are rhythms in the struggles and triumphs and the ups and downs of everyday living with others. Practicing within the theory of human becoming, the nurse does not try to change these rhythms or assist the family or individual to adapt, but moves with the rhythm, guiding individuals and families to find their own harmony within the situation, leading them to find their own meaning. The process for the nurse: "Dwelling with is giving self over to the struggle in connecting-separating" (Parse, 1987, p. 167).

Mobilizing Transcendence

The dimension of "mobilizing transcendence through moving beyond" (Parse, 1987, p. 167) flows directly from Principle 3—cotranscending with the possibles. As the nurse dwells in true presence with clients/families as they struggle with the ever-changing situations, they move beyond (transcend) the present meaning of the events in their lives "to what is not yet . . . dreaming of the possibles and planning to reach for the dreams. The nurse guides individuals and families to plan for the changing of lived health patterns—these patterns uncovered in the illuminating of meaning, synchronizing of rhythms, and mobilizing of transcendence" (Parse, 1987, p. 169).

6

Clinical Example

An excellent example of the use of Parse's theory to guide clinical practice was described by Butler (1988) in the case of an elderly hospitalized father who was confused and frightened by treatment and who begged his family to take him home. The nurse, rather than attempting to orient the father or advise the family, guided them through the process of finding their own meaning in the situation (illuminating meaning through explicating). The nurse posed questions to the family and helped them clarify their thoughts and feelings and to share these with one another. The insights gained by the new meanings were explored and the family arrived at a new consensus and connectedness. Their altered view of the situation enabled them to support the father in his refusal to have physical therapy and led them to request that his tranquilizer be discontinued. In these decisions, the family elected to move with their father's reality. The nurse, in directing energy toward the planning for this different mode, was synchronizing the rhythms of the family (as well as those of the health care agency). The nurse asked questions, clarified perceptions, pointed out and explored options, and helped them to learn ways of taking care of the father in the daughter's home. The family, however, set their own rhythms, struggled with the responsibility of their choices, and came to live their own value priorities. The nurse neither advocated nor discredited the plan to remove the father from the hospital, but went with the rhythm of the family.

Dramatic progress was evident in the father as soon as he began to live in his daughter's home, and, within 10 days, he requested to go to his own home. Again, the nurse dwelled with the family members in the revealing-concealing of their fears and concerns about the enabling-limiting possibilities of this proposed change. The second move represented a separating from a now familiar and safe environment while connecting with the cherished desire of living in his own home with his wife. The couple's home was altered to make it safer and easier for them to care for one another and the nurse arranged to make regular visits. The father, cotranscending with the new possibles, began to unfold a new pattern of health. His physicians were amazed at the progress of his medical condition. Leaving the doctors' offices with the nurse, the father, noting that it was raining, picked up his walker and ran to the car.

Butler (1988) stated that the dimension of mobilizing transcendence by moving beyond to new possibilities was evident in all facets of the nurse's practice (see Appendix). This dimension was particularly evident when the nurse helped the family to image new possibilities and to move beyond in each of the connecting-separating instances when the father left the hospital and then his daughter's home.

Other published examples of clinical nursing practice guided by Parse's theory include the case of an elderly client who was actually in a hospital ward, but whose coconstituted reality placed her in a park (Mitchell, 1986). Being present to the client's languaging, the nurse realized the client was multidimensionally experiencing her past (childhood and young adulthood), present, and future simultaneously. The nurse did not contradict the patient's reality, but validated her feelings, guiding her to express her personal meanings and offering information and freedom to make choices. Another example of practice based on Parse's theory was an account of a nurse dwelling with a family that was cotranscending patterns of spouse abuse (Butler & Snodgrass, 1991).

7

Research Methodologies in the Theory of Human Becoming

Research Topics

The worldview and the assumptions of Parse's theory of human becoming lead the nurse to choose as the major focus for study the commonly lived experiences of human beings. Such health-related experiences include those which reflect the concepts of Parse's theory: being-becoming, value priorities, negentropic unfolding, and others relating to the quality of life for the person/family (Parse, 1987, p. 174). Examples of topics that have been studied are: *Persisting in Change Even Though It Is Difficult: The Lived Experience Of Health,* (Parse, 1985b) and *Struggling Through a Difficult Time for Unemployed Persons* (Smith, 1990).

Research Processes

Parse's is one of the few nursing theories for which a research methodology specific to the theory has been developed. The processes used to study the topics listed above connect with and are consistent with the theory. *Dialogical engagement* is the term for the discussion between participant and researcher (Parse, 1987). The researcher dwells with the ideas of the meaning of the experience and brings some questions and direction to begin the dialogue. These are not precise and predefined as in a printed questionnaire, but a sharing of the sense of the question as it has originated. The genuine direction of the dialogue emerges from the lived experience and the recounting by the participant. *Extraction-synthesis* is the process by which the researcher dwells with the transcribed dialogue, moving to higher levels of abstraction to the structure of the evolved answers to the research question, which is, "What is the structure of this lived experience?" (Parse, 1987, p. 177). The major processes utilized by the researcher are (a) extracting essences, (b) synthesizing essences, (c) formulating propositions, (d) extracting concepts, and (e) synthesizing a structure of the lived experience from the extracted concepts.

Heuristic interpretation consists of *structural integration* in which the propositions and structures are connected to the theory, and *conceptual interpretation*, which interprets the essences synthesized from the lived experiences in light of the concepts of Parse's theory. These processes lead to the formulation of specific theoretical structures derived from the theory. (See "Theoretical Structures," described above). "The heuristic interpretation weaves the ideas of the structure as lived into the theory and propels it beyond to posit ideas for research studies and possible practice activities" (Parse, 1987, p. 177).

Example of Research Methodology

Kelley (1991) used Parse's methodology to generate a study of the lived experience of "struggling with going along in a situation you do not believe in." Following Parse's guidelines, the researcher centered on the meaning of the phenomenon and then made herself authentically present to the study participants in dialogical engagement, allowing their experiences to emerge in the open interviews. The researcher then spent time listening intensively to the tapes and reading the transcripts, dwelling with the data to extract essences, or core ideas, and synthesizing these essences at a higher level of abstraction. Propositions were formulated for each participant, and core concepts for the group were extracted. The concepts were then synthesized into a structure of the lived experience. Core concepts identified by Kelley were (a) justifiable yielding, (b) opposing views intensifying personal convictions, and (c) compelled disclosure while suffering consequences (Kelley, 1991, p. 127). *Structural integration*, defined as connecting the structure of the lived experience with the theory, raised the abstraction of the concepts to (a) choosing priorities, (b) pushing-resisting, and (c) disclosing-not disclosing. The conceptual interpretation of these within Parse's theory was (a) valuing, (b) powering, and (c) revealing-concealing, or "struggling with going along in a situation you do not believe in is valuing the powering of revealing-concealing" (Kelley, 1991, p. 128).

The emerging methodology briefly described here differs from other methods used in nursing research. Because it focuses on the lived experiences of human beings, Parse presented it as an appropriate methodology to study the phenomena of interest to nurses.

8

Conclusion

Parse's theory of human becoming is important in its position among nursing theories that strive to provide the profession with guidelines for nursing practice, research, and education in a new age. It offers assumptions that provide a new and different view of health and an insight into the participation of persons in creating their own reality, a factor that nurses have always recognized. This theory provides concepts and tools for nurses to think about and to help them work with these client realities. Firmly rooted in the human sciences, Parse's theory fits with the intuitive search for frameworks that describe what some nurses have come to believe about their discipline and profession as well as what nurses actually do in their interaction with clients. It provides a map for many of the entities that nurses are dealing with: meanings, feelings, alternate interpretations of reality, communications, and values. It is also a very useful theory in that it addresses the struggles of clients, nurses, and families to assimilate and integrate change.

Appendix: Clinical Example

Dimensions	Processes of Nurse	Processes of Family
Illuminating Meaning	Assisting family members in clarifying their ideas, sharing their thoughts	Exploring meaning of father's reality with him
		Expressing feelings including guilt, loneliness, and frustration
	Posing questions	
	Guiding the family in explicating the meaning of their current situation	Sharing feelings, values, and dreams
		Developing a consensus on new insights into the father's and family's situation (a cocreated different view)
Synchronizing Rhythms	Directing family's energy toward planning for the new possibility	Family makes a choice to go with the rhythm set by the father
		Begin to discuss how a reuniting of the family might be brought about

continued

33

Dimensions	Processes of Nurse	Processes of Family
	Helping the family explore the merits and drawbacks of all suggested possibilities	Exploring the possibilities of taking the father home
	Questioning, clarifying answers	Struggling with responsibilities and options
	Suggesting and exploring options	Devising a plan
	Neither advocating nor discrediting any plan proposed by family	Learning to perform some tasks for the father
	Going with the flow of the family's struggle to get the father home	Setting their own rhythm in devising their plan. Becoming more aware of their own and one another's values in self-disclosure (revealing-concealing)
		Coconstituting desired ways of being in the world
		Living their value priorities
Mobilizing Transcendence	Preparing family to take father home	Family members move toward a clear understanding of the situation and one another
	Moving beyond at each level with the family	
	Being with the family as they struggle with familiar and unfamiliar patterns in finding new ways of being	Each member changes and the family struggles to find new ways of being together
		They achieve their goal of making their father comfortable in his own home

continued

Dimensions	Processes of Nurse	Processes of Family
	Helping the family to be with the cherished familiar in new ways by exploring options, listening to ideas, analyzing viewpoints	They create a new emergence by inventing different ways of living their values

SOURCE: Butler (1988).

Glossary

Coconstitution
The human being's "active participation in creating meaning with others and the world" (Parse, 1981, p. 177).

Cocreate
"Initiate anew with another; coconstitute" (Parse, 1981, p. 177).

Cotranscending
"Going beyond the actual in interrelationship with others" (Parse, 1987, p. 166).

Health
"Process of becoming as experienced and described by the person" (Parse, 1992, p. 36). "Health is man's patterns of relating value priorities . . . an intersubjective process of transcending with the possibles" (Parse, 1981, p. 33). "Health is Man's unfolding. It is Man's lived experiences, a nonlinear entity that is not qualified or quantified by terms such as good, bad, more, or less. It is not Man adapting or coping. Unitary Man's health is a synthesis of values, a way of living. It is not the opposite of disease or a state that man has, but rather is a continuously changing process that Man cocreates." (Parse, 1987, p. 160). "Health is an expression of values at the moment, the meaning given to a situation" (Parse, 1987, p. 163). "It is just the way the human is! Health is cocreated through the human-environment interrelationship, and it is lived in rhythmical

patterns of relating that incarnate the meaning that the human being gives to situations" (Parse, 1990, p. 137).

Helicy

"Continuous, innovative, unpredictable, increasing diversity of human and environmental field patterns" (Rogers, 1990, p. 8).

Imaging

"Symbolizing or picturing" (Parse, 1981, p. 177). "Imaging refers to knowing; exists at the explicit and tacit realms" (Parse, 1992, p. 37).

Integrality

"Continuous mutual human field and environmental field process" (Rogers, 1990, p. 8). Formerly termed *complementary*.

Intersubjectivity

Subject-to-subject relationship involving true presence (Parse, 1981, p. 177).

Knowing

"Personal knowledge is shaped through prereflective-reflective imaging, explicitly and tacitly all at once. Explicit knowing is reflected upon critically; tacit knowing is prearticulate and acritical" (Parse, 1992, p. 37).

Languaging

"Sharing valued images through symbols of words, gesture, gaze, touch, and posture" (Parse, 1981, p. 177). It "is the way human beings represent personal structures of reality" (Parse, 1992, p. 37).

Man

"Refers to *homo sapiens*" (Parse, 1981, p. xiii). "Man is an open being, more than and different from the sum of parts in mutual simultaneous interchange with the environment who chooses from options and bears responsibility for choices. Man cocreates patterns of relating with the environment and is recognized by these patterns" (Parse, 1987, p. 160). "Man is coexisting while coconstituting rhythmical patterns with the environment . . . Man is transcending multidimensionally with the possibles" (Parse, 1981, p. 33).

Man-living-health

"A unitary phenomenon that refers to man's becoming through cocreating rhythmical patterns of relating in open energy interchange with the environment" (Parse, 1981, p. 39). This combination of words with their hyphens indicates one concept with a meaning different from the separate words. The phrase *man-living-health* indicates "health as ongoing participation with the world" (Parse, 1981, p. 39).

Multidimensionally
"Refers to the various levels of the universe that Man experiences all at once. Specifically the term refers to explicit-tacit knowing. Not all choices are made from the explicit level. Man chooses possibilities from the whole sense of the situation. With each situation there are multiple possibles unfolding. What unfolds surfaces in relationship to others and the environment as dreams of what can be become actualities" (Parse, 1987, pp. 161-162).

Originating
"Creating anew, generating unique ways of living which surface through interconnections with people and projects" (Parse, 1992, p. 38).

Paradigm
"A way of viewing a particular field of study" (Parse, 1981, p. 178).

Paradox
"Refers to apparent opposites. These rhythmical patterns are not opposites; they are two sides of the same rhythm that coexist all at once" (Parse, 1992, p. 38).

Pattern
"A configuration of man-environment interrelationship" (Parse, 1981, p. 178).

Phenomenology
"The study of phenomena as they unfold" (Parse, 1981, p. 178).

Possibles
"The imaginables toward which one reaches" (Parse, 1981, p. 178).

Powering
"Is the pushing-resisting rhythm in all and human-universe inter-relationships. It is the back and forth experienced by humans in all life situations, an energizing force which sparks moving beyond the moment" (Parse, 1992, p. 38).

Theoretical structures

"A statement interrelating concepts in a way that can be verified" (Parse, 1981, p. 179). "Nondirectional propositions," statements that are "noncausal in nature and consistent with the assumptions and principles [of Parse's theory]." "They are designed to guide practice and research." (Parse, 1987, p. 166). "To make these usable in practice and research, statements about nursing practice must be derived and lived experiences chosen for study" (Parse, 1987, p. 166).

Transcending

"Going beyond; exceeding" (Parse, 1981, p. 179).

Transforming

"The shifting of views of the familiar as different light is shed on what is known. Change itself is a continuous ongoing process in the human-universe process which is recognized by increasing diversity" (Parse, 1992, p. 39).

Valuing

"The process of living cherished beliefs while assimilating the new into a personal worldview. It emerges in the human-universe process and is the human being's confirming of cherished beliefs" (Parse, 1992, p. 37).

Wholeness

"More than and different from the sum of parts" (Parse, 1981, p. 179).

References

Butler, M. J. (1988). Family transformation: Parse's theory in practice. *Nursing Science Quarterly, 1,* 68-74.

Butler, M. J., & Snodgrass, F. G. (1991). Beyond abuse: Parse's theory in practice. *Nursing Science Quarterly, 4,* 76-82.

Heidegger, M. (1962). *Being and time.* New York: Harper & Row.

Kelley, L. S. (1991). Struggling with going along when you do not believe. *Nursing Science Quarterly, 4*(3), 123-129.

Lavine, T. Z. (1984). *From Socrates to Sartre: The philosophic quest.* New York: Bantam.

Lee, R. E., & Schumacher, L. P. (1989). Rosemarie Rizzo Parse. In A. Marriner-Tomey (Ed.), *Nursing theorists and their work* (2nd ed., pp. 174-186). St. Louis: Mosby.

Merleau-Ponty, M. (1962). *Phenomenology of perception.* New York: The Humanities Press.

Mitchell, G. J. (1986). Utilizing Parse's theory of Man-Living-Health in Mrs. M's neighborhood. *Perspectives, 10*(4), 5-7.

Mitchell, G. J., & Santopinto, M. (1988). An alternative to nursing diagnosis. *The Canadian Nurse, 84*(10), 25-28.

Parse, R. R. (1974). *Nursing fundamentals.* Flushing, NY: Medical Examination.

Parse, R. R. (1981). *Man-Living-Health: A theory of nursing.* New York: John Wiley.

Parse, R. R. (Speaker). (1985a). *Presentation at nurse theorist conference.* (Cassette Recording No. DII-105). Louisville, KY: Meetings Internationale.

Parse, R. R. (1985b). Nursing research traditions quantitative and qualitative approaches. In R. R. Parse, A. B. Coyne, & M. J. Smith (Eds.), *Nursing research qualitative methods* (pp. 1-8). Bowie, MD: Brady Communications.

Parse, R. R. (1987). Man-Living-Health theory of nursing. In R. R. Parse (Ed.), *Nursing science: Major paradigms, theories and critiques* (pp. 159-180). Philadelphia: W. B. Saunders.

Parse, R. R. (1990). Health: A personal commitment. *Nursing Science Quarterly,* 3(3), 136-140.

Parse, R. R. (1992). Human becoming: Parse's theory of nursing. *Nursing Science Quarterly,* 5(1), 35-42.

Rogers, M. E. (1970). *An introduction to the theoretical basis of nursing.* Philadelphia: F. A. Davis.

Rogers, M. E. (1980). Nursing: A science of unitary man. In J. P. Riehl & C. Roy (Eds.), *Conceptual models for nursing practice* (2nd ed., pp. 329-337). New York: Appleton-Century-Crofts.

Rogers, M. E. (1987). Rogers's science of unitary human beings. In R. R. Parse (Ed.), *Nursing science: Major paradigms, theories, and critiques* (pp. 139-146). Philadelphia: W. B. Saunders.

Rogers, M. E. (1990). Nursing: Science of unitary, irreducible, human beings: Update 1990. In E. A. M. Barrett (Ed.), *Visions of Rogers's science-based nursing* (pp. 5-11). New York: National League for Nursing.

Sartre, J. P. (1956). *Being and nothingness.* New York: Washington Square.

Smith, M. C. (1990). Struggling through a difficult time for unemployed persons. *Nursing Science Quarterly, 3,* 18-28.

Smith, M. C., & Hudepohl, J. H. (1988). Analysis and evaluation of Parse's theory of Man-Living-Health. *Canadian Journal of Nursing Research, 20*(4), 43-58.

Bibliography:
References Related to Parse's Work

Primary Sources

Books

Parse, R. R. (1974). *Nursing fundamentals*. Flushing, NY: Medical Examination.

Parse, R. R. (1981). *Man-living-health: A theory of nursing*. New York: John Wiley.

Parse, R. R. (1987). *Nursing science: Major paradigms, theories, and critiques*. Philadelphia: W. B. Saunders.

Parse, R. R., Coyne, A. B., & Smith, M. J. (1985). *Nursing research: Qualitative methods*. Bowie, MD: Robert J. Brady.

Doctoral Dissertation

Parse, R. R. (1969). An instructional model for the teaching of nursing, interrelating objectives and media (Doctoral dissertation, University of Pittsburgh). *Dissertation Abstracts International, 31*, 180A.

Book Chapters, Articles, and Editorials

Parse, R. R. (1967, August). The advantages of the ADN program. *Journal of Nursing Education, 6*(15).

Parse, R. R. (1978). Rights of medical patients. In C. Fisher (Ed.), *Client participation in human services*. New Brunswick, NJ: Transaction.

Parse, R. R. (1980). Caring from a human science perspective. In M. M. Leininger (Ed.), *Caring: A human helping process*. Salt Lake City, UT.

Parse, R. R. (1981). Caring from a human science perspective. In M. M. Leininger (Ed.), *Caring: An essential human need*. Thorofare, NJ: Charles B. Slack.

Parse, R. R. (1988). Beginnings. *Nursing Science Quarterly, 1,* 1.

Parse, R. R. (1988). Creating traditions: The art of putting it together. *Nursing Science Quarterly 1,* 45.

Parse, R. R. (1988). Scholarly dialogue: The fire of refinement. *Nursing Science Quarterly, 1,* 141.

Parse, R. R. (1988). The mainstream of science: Framing the issue. *Nursing Science Quarterly, 1,* 93.

Parse, R. R. (1989). Essentials for practicing the art of nursing. *Nursing Science Quarterly, 2,* 111.

Parse, R. R. (1989). Making more out of less. *Nursing Science Quarterly, 2,* 155.

Parse, R. R. (1989). Man-living-health: A theory of nursing. In J. Riehl-Sisca (Ed.), *Conceptual models for nursing practice* (3rd ed.). Norwalk, CT: Appleton & Lange.

Parse, R. R. (1989). Martha E. Rogers: A birthday celebration. *Nursing Science Quarterly, 2,* 55.

Parse, R. R. (1989). Parse's man-living-health model and administration of nursing services. In B. Henry, C. Arndt, M. DiVincenti, & A. Marriner-Tomey (Eds.), *Dimensions of nursing administration: Theory, research, education, and practice*. Cambridge, MA: Blackwell Scientific Publications.

Parse, R. R. (1989). Qualitative research: Publishing and funding. *Nursing Science Quarterly, 2,* 1.

Parse, R. R. (1989). The phenomenological research method: Its value for management science. In B. Henry, C. Arndt, M. DiVincenti, & A. Marriner Tomey (Eds.), *Dimensions of nursing administration: Theory, research, education, and practice*. Cambridge, MA: Blackwell Scientific Publications.

Parse, R. R. (1990). A time for reflection and projection. *Nursing Science Quarterly, 3,* 141-143.

Parse, R. R. (1990). Health: A personal commitment. *Nursing Science Quarterly, 3,* 136-140.

Parse, R. R. (1990). Nurse theorist conference comes to Japan. *Japanese Journal of Nursing Research, 23*(3).

Parse, R. R. (1990). Nursing theory-based practice: A challenge for the 90s. *Nursing Science Quarterly, 3,* 53.

Parse, R. R. (1990). Parse's research methodology with an illustration of the lived experience of hope. *Nursing Science Quarterly, 3,* 9-17.

Parse, R. R. (1990). Promotion and prevention: Two distinct cosmologies. *Nursing Science Quarterly, 3,* 101.

Parse, R. R. (1991). Electronic publishing: Beyond browsing. *Nursing Science Quarterly, 4,* 1.

Parse, R. R. (1991). Growing: The discipline of nursing. *Nursing Science Quarterly, 4,* 139.

Parse, R. R. (1991). Mysteries of health and healing: Two perspectives. *Nursing Science Quarterly, 4,* 93.

Parse, R. R. (1991). Phenomenology and nursing. *Japanese Journal of Nursing, 17*(2), 261-269.

Parse, R. R. (1991). The right soil, the right stuff. *Nursing Science Quarterly, 4,* 47.
Parse, R. R. (in press). Man-living-health: A theory of nursing. In M. Mischo-Kelling & K. Wittneben (Eds.), *Auffassungen von Pflege in theorie und praxis.*

Unpublished Manuscripts (past 4 years)

Parse, R. R. (1987). *Man-living-health and the meaning of aging.* Paper presented at Gerontological Society Meeting, Washington, DC.
Parse, R. R. (1988). *Nursing science: The development and testing of theory.* Keynote address at Southern Council on Collegiate Education for Nursing Research conference, Atlanta.
Parse, R. R. (1988). *Parse's theory, research and practice.* Paper presented at Annual Doctoral Students Research Conference, Wayne State University, School of Nursing, Detroit.
Parse, R. R. (1988). *Parse's theory in practice: An evaluation study.* Paper presented at National Symposium of Nursing Research, San Francisco.
Parse, R. R. (1989). *Nursing as a discipline: Its theories and methods of inquiry.* SUNY Downstate, NY.
Parse, R. R. (1989). *Parse's theory of nursing.* Cedars Medical Center Nursing Theory Conference, Miami, FL.
Parse, R. R. (1989). *Publications in scholarly journals.* ANA Council of Nurse Researchers, Chicago.
Parse, R. R. (1989). *Qualitative research: The new story in sciencing.* Keynote address, Barry University, University of Miami and South Florida Nursing Research Society, Miami.
Parse, R. R. (1989). Symposium for doctoral students and faculty on research and theory development, simultaneity paradigm, Medical College of Georgia, Augusta.
Parse, R. R. (1989). *The quest for knowledge: Imagining, enlightening, enlivening.* Barry University 50th Jubilee, Miami Shores, FL.
Parse, R. R. (1989). *Using nursing knowledge in practice.* Keynote address, Cedars Medical Center Nursing Theory Conference, Miami, FL.
Parse, R. R. *Research methods unique to nursing.* Keynote address, Barry University, University of Miami and South Florida Nursing Research Society, Miami.
Parse, R. R. (1990). *A dialogue with nurse theorists: A basis for differentiating nursing practice.* Paper presented at American Academy of Nursing, Charleston, SC.
Parse, R. R. (1990). *Advancing nursing science through qualitative research.* Paper presented at Eastern Nursing Research Society, New York.
Parse, R. R. (1990). *Man-living-health: Theory, research and practice.* Paper presented at University of South Carolina, College of Nursing, Columbia.
Parse, R. R. (1990). *Man-living-health theory and the meaning of health and cultural values in elders.* Paper presented at 43rd Annual Scientific Session, The Gerontological Society of America, Boston.
Parse, R. R. (1990). *Parse's research and practice methodologies.* Paper presented at Discovery International, Inc., Nursing Science Seminar, Vernon Manor Hotel, Cincinnati, OH.

Parse, R. R. (1990). *Parse's theory: A way of living nursing.* Paper presented at The Queen Elizabeth Hospital, Nursing Division, Toronto, Ontario.

Parse, R. R. (1990). *Parse's theory in practice: A workshop.* Presented at North Shore Medical Center, Miami, FL.

Parse, R. R. (1990). *Parse's theory in practice and research.* Paper presented at Sigma Theta Tau, Alpha Phi Chapter, Annual Research Day, Hunter-Bellevue School of Nursing, New York.

Parse, R. R. (1990). *Parse's theory in research and practice.* UCLA Neuro-Psychiatric Institute and Hospital, Nursing Department, Los Angeles.

Parse, R. R. (1990). *Qualitative research.* Paper presented at University of South Carolina, College of Nursing, Columbia.

Parse, R. R. (1990). *Reporting research: From article to abstract.* Paper presented at Teachers College Columbia University, New York, NY.

Parse, R. R. (1990). *Simultaneity paradigm and Parse's theory.* Paper presented at University of Pittsburgh, Pittsburgh.

Parse, R. R. (1990). *The meaning of choosing health.* Paper presented at Harmarville Rehabilitation Center, Harmarville, PA.

Parse, R. R. (1991). *Man-living health, theory, research and practice.* Paper presented at Kyoto, Japan.

Parse, R. R. (1991). *Nursing knowledge for the 21st century: An international commitment.* Keynote address at Discovery International, Inc., Biennial Nurse Theorist Conference, Tokyo, Japan.

Parse, R. R. (1991). *Nursing theory-based practice: Does it make a difference?* Paper presented at Battle Creek Veteran's Administration Medical Center Conference, Kalamazoo, MI.

Parse, R. R. (1991). *Parse in question and answer.* Discovery International, Inc., Biennial Nurse Theorist Conference, Tokyo, Japan.

Parse, R. R. (1991). *Parse's human becoming theory of nursing.* Paper presented at Battle Creek Veteran's Administration Medical Center Conference, Kalamazoo, MI.

Parse, R. R. (1991). *Parse's theory.* Paper presented at Discovery International, Inc., Biennial Nurse Theorist Conference, Tokyo, Japan.

Parse, R. R. (1991). *Phenomenology as a way of living.* Paper presented at Interpersonal Relationships Society, Tokyo, Japan.

Parse, R. R. (1991). *Theory and research as tools for practice.* Paper presented at University of Michigan, School of Nursing, Centennial Celebration, Ann Arbor.

Cassette Recordings

Parse, R. R. (Speaker). (1985). *Nursing education in the 21st century.* (Cassette Recording No. DII-113). Louisville, KY: Meetings Internationale.

Parse, R. R. (Speaker). (1985). *Presentation at nurse theorist conference.* (Cassette Recording No. DII-105). Louisville, KY: Meetings Internationale.

Parse, R. R., Orem, D. E., Roy, D., King, I. M., Rogers, M. E., & Peplau, H. E. (Speakers). (1985). *Panel discussion with nurse theorists.* (Cassette Recording No. DII-112). Louisville, KY: Meetings Internationale.

Parse, R. R., & Phillips, J. R. (Speakers). (1985). *Parse's man-living-health theory of nursing*. (Cassette Recording No. DII-109). Louisville, KY: Meetings Internationale.

Parse, R. R. (Speaker). (1986). *An emerging research methodology unique to nursing*. (Cassette Recording No. DII-303). Louisville, KY: Meetings Internationale.

Parse, R. R. (Speaker). (1986). *Panel discussion*. (Cassette Recording No. DII-305). Louisville, KY: Meetings Internationale.

Parse, R. R. (Speaker). (1986). *Quantitative and qualitative methods in nursing research*. (Cassette Recording No. DII-201). Louisville, KY: Meetings Internationale.

Parse, R. R. (Speaker). (1986). *The ethnographic method*. (Cassette Recording No. DII-204). Louisville, KY: Meetings Internationale.

Parse, R. R. (Speaker). (1986). *The phenomenological method*. (Cassette Recording No. DII-202[A&B]). Louisville, KY: Meetings Internationale.

Parse, R. R. (Speaker). (1987). *Panel discussion with theorists*. (Cassette Recording No. DII-408). Louisville, KY: Meetings Internationale.

Parse, R. R. (Speaker). (1987). *Parse's theory*. (Cassette Recording No. DII-403). Louisville, KY: Meetings Internationale.

Parse, R. R. (Speaker). (1987). *Small group C*. (Cassette Recording No. DII-411). Louisville, KY: Meetings Internationale.

Parse, R. R. (Speaker). (1989). *Health as a personal commitment in Parse's theory*. (Cassette Recording No. DII-503). Louisville, KY: Meetings Internationale.

Parse, R. R. (Speaker). (1989). *Panel discussion with theorists*. (Cassette Recording No. DII-507). Louisville, KY: Meetings Internationale.

Parse, R. R. (Speaker). (1990). *Panel discussion/retrospective and evaluation*. (Cassette Recording No. DII-605). Louisville, KY: Meetings Internationale.

Parse, R. R. (Speaker). (1990). *Parse's research and practice methodologies*. (Cassette Recording No. DII-601). Louisville, KY: Meetings Internationale.

Videotape Recordings

Parse, R. R., Orem, D. E., Roy, C., King, I. M., Rogers, M. E., & Peplau, H. E. (Speakers). (1985). *Panel discussion with theorists*. (Videotape Recording No. DII-V-112). Louisville, KY: Meetings Internationale.

Parse, R. R. (Speaker). (1987). *Parse's theory*. (Videotape Recording No. DII-V-403). Louisville, KY: Meetings Internationale.

Parse, R. R., Peplau, H. E., King, I. M., Roy, C., Rogers, M. E., Watson, J., & Leininger, M. (Speakers). (1987). *Panel discussion with theorists*. (Videotape Recording No. DII-V-408). Louisville, KY: Meetings Internationale.

Parse, R. R. (Speaker). (1989). *Health as a personal commitment in Parse's theory*. (Videotape Recording No. DII-V-503). Louisville, KY: Meetings Internationale.

Parse, R. R., Meleis, A. I., Neuman, B. M., Rogers, M. E., Pender, N. J., & King., I. M. (Speakers). (1989). *Panel discussion with theorists*. (Videotape Recording No. DII-V-507). Louisville, KY: Meetings Internationale.

Parse, R. R. (Speaker). (1990). *A portrait in excellence* [Videotape]. Helene Fuld Health Trust. Oakland, CA: Studio Three Production.

Secondary Sources

Book Reviews on Parse's Books

Parse, R. R. (1975). *Nursing fundamentals.* In *Australian Nurses Journal, 5*(37).

Parse, R. R. (1981). *Man-living-health: A theory of nursing.* In *International Journal of Rehabilitation Research, 4,* 449, and in *Western Journal of Nursing Research, 5,* 105-106, Winter 1982.

Parse, R. R., Coyne, A. B., & Smith, M. J. (1986). *Nursing research: Qualitative methods.* Review of four general nursing research methods tests. By E. R. Lenz in *Nursing Science Quarterly, 1,* 86-90.

Parse, R. R. (1988). *Nursing science: Major paradigms, theories, and critiques.* Three perspectives on a scholarly work. By M. K. Jacobs-Kramer, M. E. Levine, & E. M. Menke in *Nursing Science Quarterly, 1,* 182-186.

Books and Articles Mentioning Parse's Theory

Chinn, P. L., & Jacobs, M. K. (1987). *Theory and nursing: A systematic approach* (2nd ed.). St. Louis: Mosby.

Fitzpatrick, J. J., & Whall, A. L. (1989). *Conceptual models of nursing: Analysis and application* (2nd ed.). Norwalk, CT: Appleton & Lange.

George, J. (1990). *Nursing theories: The base for professional nursing practice* (3rd ed.). New York: Prentice Hall.

Kleffel, D. (1991). Rethinking the environment as a domain of nursing knowledge. *Advances in Nursing Science, 14,* 10-51.

Marriner-Tomey, A. (1989). *Nursing theorists and their work* (2nd ed.). St. Louis: Mosby.

Meleis, A. I. (1985). *Theoretical nursing: Development and progress.* Philadelphia: J. B. Lippincott.

Mitchell, G. J. (1991). Nursing diagnosis: An ethical analysis. *Image: Journal of Nursing Scholarship, 23,* 99-103.

Nagle, L. M., & Mitchell, G. J. (1991). Theoretic diversity: Evolving paradigmatic issues in research and practice. *Advances in Nursing Science, 14,* 17-25.

Newman, M. A., Sime, A. M., & Corcoran-Perry, S. A. (1991). The focus of the discipline of nursing. *Advances in Nursing Science, 14,* 1-6.

Book Chapters and Articles by Others on Parse

Cowling, W. R. (1989). Parse's theory of nursing. In J. J. Fitzpatrick & A. L. Whall (Eds.), *Conceptual models of nursing: Analysis and application,* (2nd ed., pp. 385-399). Norwalk, CT: Appleton & Lange.

Hickman, J. S. (1990). Rosemarie Rizzo Parse. In J. B. George (Ed.), *Nursing theories: The base for professional nursing practice* (3rd ed., pp. 311-332). Norwalk, CT: Appleton & Lange.

Lee, R. E., & Schumacher, L. P. (1989). Rosemarie Rizzo Parse: Man-living-health. In A. Marriner-Tomey (Ed.), *Nurse theorists and their work* (2nd ed., pp. 174-186). St. Louis, MO: Mosby.

Phillips, J. (1987). A critique of Parse's man-living-health theory. In R. R. Parse, *Nursing science: Major paradigms, theories and critiques* (pp. 181-204). Philadelphia: W. B. Saunders.

Pugliese, L. (1989). The theory of man-living-health: An analysis. In J. Riehl-Sisca (Ed.), *Conceptual models for nursing practice* (3rd ed., pp. 259-265). Norwalk, CT: Appleton & Lange.

Smith, M. C., & Hudepohl, J. H. (1988). Analysis and evaluation of Parse's theory of man-living-health. *The Canadian Journal of Nursing Research: Nursing Papers, 20*(4), 43-58.

Winkler, S. J. (1983). Parse's theory of nursing. In J. J. Fitzpatrick & A. L. Whall (Eds.), *Conceptual models of nursing: Analysis and application* (pp. 275-294). Bowie, MD: Robert J. Brady.

Directories and Biographical Sources

Fellow in the American Academy of Nursing. (1989). *Directory of Fellows in AAN*.

Sigma Theta Tau. (1987). *Directory of nurse researchers* (2nd ed.). Indianapolis, IN.

Articles About Parse's Theory

Banonis, B. C. (1989). The lived experience of recovering from addiction: A phenomenological study. *Nursing Science Quarterly, 2*, 37-43.

Butler, M. J. (1988). Family transformation: Parse's theory in practice. *Nursing Science Quarterly, 1*, 68-74.

Butler, M. J., & Snodgrass, F. G. (1991). Beyond abuse: Parse's theory in practice. *Nursing Science Quarterly, 4*, 76-82.

Cody, W. K. (in press). Grieving a personal loss. *Nursing Science Quarterly, 4*, 61-68.

Heine, C. (1991). Development of gerontological nursing theory: Applying man-living-health theory of nursing. *Nursing & Health Care, 12*, 184-188.

Kelley, L. M. (1991). Struggling with going along when you do not believe. *Nursing Science Quarterly, 4*, 123-129.

Liehr, P. R. (1989). The core of true presence: A loving center. *Nursing Science Quarterly, 2*, 7-8.

Mattice, M. (1991). Parse's theory of nursing in practice: A manager's perspective. *The Canadian Journal of Nursing Administration*, 11-13.

Mattice, M., & Mitchell, G. J. (1991). Caring for confused elders. *The Canadian Nurse, 86*(11), 16-17.

Mitchell, G. J. (1986). Utilizing Parse's theory of man-living-health in Mrs. M's neighborhood. *Perspectives, 10*(4), 5-7.

Mitchell, G. J. (1988). Man-living-health: The theory in practice. *Nursing Science Quarterly, 1*, 120-127.

Mitchell G. J. (1990). Struggling in change: From the traditional approach to Parse's theory-based practice. *Nursing Science Quarterly, 3*, 170-176.

Mitchell, G. J. (1990). The lived experience of taking life day-by-day in later life: Research guided by Parse's emergent method. *Nursing Science Quarterly, 3*, 29-36.

Mitchell, G. J. (1991). Diagnosis: Clarifying or obscuring the nature of nursing. *Nursing Science Quarterly, 4,* 52-53.

Mitchell, G. J. (1991). Nursing diagnosis: An ethical analysis. *Image: Journal of Nursing Scholarship.*

Mitchell, G. J., & Copplestone, C. (1990). Applying Parse's theory to perioperative nursing: A nontraditional approach. *AORN Journal, 51*(3), 787-798.

Mitchell, G. J., & Pilkington, B. (1990). Theoretical approaches in nursing practice: A comparison of Roy and Parse. *Nursing Science Quarterly, 3,* 81-87.

Mitchell, G. J., & Santopinto, M. D. A. (1988). An alternative to nursing diagnosis. *The Canadian Nurse, 84*(10), 25-28.

Mitchell, G. J., & Santopinto, M. D. A. (1988). The expanded role nurse: A dissenting viewpoint. *The Canadian Journal of Nursing Administration, 4*(1), 8-14.

Nokes, K. M., & Carver, K. (1991). The meaning of living with AIDS: A study of using Parse's theory of man-living-health. *Nursing Science Quarterly, 4,* 174-179.

Quiquero, A., Knights, D., & Meo, C. O. (1991). Theory as a guide to practice: Staff nurses choose Parse's theory. *The Canadian Journal for Nursing Administration,* 14-16.

Rasmusson, D., Jonas, C. M., & Mitchell, G. J. (in press). The eye of the beholder: Applying Parse's theory with homeless individuals. *Clinical Nurse Specialist Journal.*

Santopinto, M. D. A. (1989). The relentless drive to be ever thinner: A study using the phenomenological method. *Nursing Science Quarterly, 2,* 29-36.

Smith, M. C. (1990). Struggling through a difficult time for unemployed persons. *Nursing Science Quarterly, 2,* 29-36.

Smith, M. J. (1989). Research and practice application related to man-living-health. In J. Riehl-Sisca (Ed.), *Conceptual models for nursing practice* (3rd ed., pp. 267-276). Norwalk, CT: Appleton & Lange.

Wondolowski, C., & Davis, D. K. (1988). The lived experience of aging in the oldest old: A phenomenological study. *The American Journal of Psychoanalysis, 48,* 261-270.

Wondolowski, C., & Davis, D. K. (1991). The lived experience of health in the oldest old: A phenomenological study. *Nursing Science Quarterly, 4,* 113-118.

Unpublished Manuscripts

Banonis, B. (1989). *The lived experience of recovering from addiction: A phenomenological study.* Paper presented at UCLA National Nursing Theory Conference, Los Angeles.

Beauchamp, C. J. (1990). *The lived experience of struggling with making a decision in a critical life situation.* Paper presented at Discovery International, Inc., Nursing Science Seminar, Research and Practice Related to Parse's Theory of Nursing, Cincinnati, OH.

Cody, W. K. (1990). *Parse's theory in practice with a grieving family.* Paper presented at Sigma Theta Tau, Alpha Phi Chapter, Annual Research Day, Hunter-Bellevue School of Nursing, New York.

Cody, W. K. (1990). *The lived experience of grieving a personal loss.* Paper presented at Discovery International, Inc., Nursing Science Seminar, Research and Practice Related to Parse's Theory of Nursing, Cincinnati, OH.

Cody, W. K. (1990). *The lived experience of grieving a personal loss.* Paper presented at UCLA National Nursing Theory Conference, Los Angeles.

Jonas, C. (1989). *Parse's theory: Research and practice.* Paper presented at the University of Toronto, School of Nursing, Ontario.

Jonas, C. (1989). *Parse's theory in practice with older people.* Paper presented at St. Michael's Hospital, Toronto, Ontario.

Jonas, C. (1989). *The lived experience of being an elder in Nepal.* Research study presented at the World Congress on Gerontology, Acapulco, Mexico.

Jonas, C. (1990). *Practicing Parse's theory with groups of individuals in the community.* Paper presented at The Queen Elizabeth Hospital, Toronto, Ontario.

Kelley, L. S. (1989). *The lived experience of "struggling with going along in a situation you do not believe in": Using the man-living-health methodology.* Paper presented at conference sponsored by Barry University, School of Nursing, Honor Society, Sigma Theta Tau, Beta Tau Chapter, University of Miami, and South Florida Nursing Research Society.

Kelley, L. S. (1990). *The lived experience of "struggling with going along in a situation you do not believe in": Using the man-living-health methodology.* Paper presented at UCLA National Nursing Theory Conference, Los Angeles.

Liehr, P. R. (1988, December). *A study of the experience of "living on the edge."* Research study presented at the Southern Council on Collegiate Education for Nursing, Atlanta.

Mattice, M. (1990). *Evaluating Parse's theory in practice.* Paper presented at the Queen Elizabeth Hospital, Toronto, Ontario.

Menke, E. M. (1990). *Critique of the research studies and the research methodology.* Paper presented at Discovery International, Inc., Nursing Science Seminar, Research and Practice Related to Parse's Theory of Nursing, Cincinnati, OH.

Misselwitz, S. K. (1989). *A phenomenological study of getting through the day for women who are homeless.* Research study presented at conference sponsored by Barry University, School of Nursing, Honor Society, Sigma Theta Tau, Beta Tau Chapter, University of Miami, and South Florida Nursing Research Society.

Mitchell, G. J. (1987). *Man-living-health in practice with the elderly.* Paper presented at Gerontological Society meeting, Washington, DC.

Mitchell, G. J. (1988). *Man-living-health in practice.* Paper presented at Wayne State University Summer Research Symposium, Detroit.

Mitchell, G. J. (1990). *A dialogue with nurse theorists: A basis for differentiating nursing practice - Parse in practice.* Paper presented at American Academy of Nursing Conference, Charleston, SC.

Mitchell, G. J. (1990). *An evaluation study of Parse's theory of nursing in an acute care setting.* Conducted and presented study at St. Michael's Hospital, Nursing Department, Toronto, Ontario.

Mitchell, G. J. (1990). *From traditional nursing to Parse's theory.* Paper presented at The Queen Elizabeth Hospital, Toronto, Ontario.

Mitchell, G. J. (1990). *Nursing practice guided by Parse's theory.* Paper presented at North Shore Medical Center, Miami, FL.

Mitchell, G. J. (1990). *Parse in practice.* Paper presented at UCLA National Nursing Theory Conference, Los Angeles.

Mitchell, G. J. (1990). *Parse's theory as a guide to practice.* Paper presented at discovery International, Inc., Nursing Science Seminar, Research and Practice Related to Parse's Theory of Nursing, Cincinnati, OH.

Pilkington, B. (1990). *Research guided by Parse's theory.* Paper presented at The Queen Elizabeth Hospital, Toronto, Ontario.

Rasmuson, D., Jonas, C., & Mitchell, G. J. (1990). *The eye of the beholder: Applying Parse's theory with homeless individuals.* Manuscript submitted for publication.

Santopinto, M. D. A. (1987). *Parse's theory of nursing as a base for innovative practice.* Paper presented at Hamilton psychiatric Hospital, Hamilton, Ontario.

Santopinto, M. D. A. (1988). *A qualitative evaluation study of Parse's theory in practice: What happens when theory is implemented?* Research study presented at Eighth Annual SCCEN Research Conference, Emory University, Atlanta.

Santopinto, M. D. A. (1988). *A test of Parse's theory in a gerontological setting: An evaluation study.* Research study presented at Ryerson Theory Congress, Toronto, Ontario.

Santopinto, M. D. A. (1988). *Close encounters of the theoretical kind: Three theory-based approaches.* Paper presented at Tenth Southeastern Conference of Specialists in Psychiatric-Mental Health Nursing, Asheville, NC.

Santopinto, M. D. A. (1989). *An emergent methodology study of caring about self for individuals who exercise relentlessly.* Research study presented at the Scientific Sessions of the Sigma Theta Tau Research Conference, Taipei, Taiwan.

Santopinto, M. D. A. (1989). *An evaluation study of Parse's practice methodology in a chronic care setting.* Research study presented at 19th Quadrennial Congress of the International Council of Nurses, Seoul, Korea.

Santopinto, M. D. A. (1990). *An evaluation of Parse's theory.* Paper presented at UCLA National Nursing Theory Conference, Los Angeles.

Santopinto, M. D. A. (1990). *An evaluation study of Parse's theory in practice.* Paper presented at Discovery International, Inc., Nursing Science Seminar, Research and Practice Related to Parse's Theory of Nursing, Cincinnati, OH.

Santopinto, M. D. A. (1990). *An evaluation study of Parse's theory in practice in a chronic long-term setting.* Paper presented at Battle Creek Veteran's Administration Medical Center Conference, Kalamazoo, MI.

Smith, M. C. (1990). *Speculation on Parse in nursing education.* Paper presented at The Queen Elizabeth Hospital, Toronto, Ontario.

Smith, M. C. (1990). *The lived experience of hope in families of critically ill persons.* Paper presented at UCLA National Nursing Theory Conference, Los Angeles.

Cassette Recordings

Beauchamp, C. J. (Speaker). (1990). *The lived experience of struggling with making a decision in a critical life situation.* (Cassette Recording No. DII-602). Louisville, KY: Meetings Internationale.

Cody, W. K. (Speaker). (1990). *The lived experience of grieving a personal loss.* (Cassette Recording No. DII-602). Louisville, KY: Meetings Internationale.

Menke, E. M. (Moderator). (1990). *Panel discussion/retrospective and evaluation*. (Cassette Recording No. DII-605). Louisville, KY: Meetings Internationale.

Menke, E. M. (Speaker). (1990). *Critique of the research studies and the research methodology*. (Cassette Recording No. DII-603). Louisville, KY: Meetings Internationale.

Mitchell, G. J. (Speaker). (1990). *Parse's theory as a guide to practice*. (Cassette Recording No. DII-604). Louisville, KY: Meetings Internationale.

Santopinto, M. D. A. (Speaker). (1990). *An evaluation study of Parse's theory in practice*. (Cassette Recording No. DII-604). Louisville, KY: Meetings Internationale.

Sklar, M. (Speaker). (1986). *The experience of living in a three generational family constellation: A case study*. (Cassette Recording No. DII-302). Louisville, KY: Meetings Internationale.

Smith, M. J. (Moderator). (1986). *Panel discussion of research related to Man-Living-Health: Evaluation*. (Cassette Recording No. DII-305). Louisville, KY: Meetings Internationale.

Smith, M. J. (Speaker). (1986). *The experience of being confined: A study using the emerging method*. (Cassette Recording No. DII-304). Louisville, KY: Meetings Internationale.

Smith, M. C. (Speaker). (1990). *The lived experience of struggling through difficult times*. (Cassette Recording No. DII-603). Louisville, KY: Meetings Internationale.

Theses and Dissertations Using Parse's Theory

Beauchamp, C. (1990). *The lived experience of struggling with making a decision in a critical life situation*. Unpublished doctoral dissertation, University of Miami, FL.

Brunsman, C. S. (1988). *A phenomenological study of the lived experience of hope in families with chronically ill children*. Unpublished master's thesis, Michigan State University, Lansing.

Cody, W. K. (1989). *Grieving a personal loss: A preliminary investigation of parse's man-living-health methodology*. Unpublished master's thesis, Hunter College, The City University of New York.

Dowling, T. C. (1987). *Sharing who you really are with another: A phenomenological inquiry*. Unpublished master's thesis, Hunter College, The City University of New York.

Huckshorn, K. A. (1988). *The lived experience of creating a new way of being*. Unpublished master's thesis, Florida State University, Tallahassee.

Nickitas, D. M. (1989). *The lived experience of choosing among life goals: A phenomenological study*. Unpublished doctoral dissertation, Adelphi University, Garden City, NY.

Petras, E. M. (1986). *The lived experience of sharing a painful moment with someone close: A phenomenological study*. Unpublished master's thesis, Hunter College, The City University of New York.

Santopinto, M. D. A. (1987). *The relentless drive to be ever thinner: A phenomenological study*. Unpublished master's thesis, The University of Western Ontario, London, Ontario.

Sklar, M. B. (1985). *Qualitative investigation of the health patterns lived in an intergenerational family lifestyle.* Unpublished master's thesis, Hunter College, The City University of New York.

Authors Citing Parse's Works

Batra, C. (1987). Nursing theory for undergraduates. *Nursing Outlook, 35*(4), 189-192.

Boyd, C. O. (1989). Dialogue on a research issue: Phenomenological research in nursing—response. *Nursing Science Quarterly, 2,* 16-19.

Boyd, C. O. (1990). Critical appraisal of developing nursing research methods. *Nursing Science Quarterly, 3,* 42-43.

Campbell, J. (1986). A survivor group for battered women. *Advances in Nursing Science, 8*(2), 13-20.

Cohen, M. Z. (1987). A historical overview of the phenomenological movement. *Image, 19*(1), 31-34.

Counts, M. M., & Boyle, J. S. (1987). Nursing, health, and policy within a community context. *Advances in Nursing Science, 9*(3), 12-23.

Cull-Willby, B. L., & Pepin, J. I. (1987). Toward a co-existence of paradigms in nursing knowledge development. *Journal of Advanced Nursing, 12*(4), 515-521.

DeFeo, D. J. (1990). Change: A central concern in nursing. *Nursing Science Quarterly, 3,* 88-94.

Duffy, M. E. (1986). Qualitative research: An approach whose time has come. *Nursing and Health Care, 7*(5), 237-239.

Gortner, S. R., & Schultz, P. R. (1988). Approaches to nursing science methods. *Image, 20*(1), 22-24.

Haase, J. E. (1987). Components of courage in chronically ill adolescents: A phenomenological study. *Advances in Nursing Science, 9*(2), 64-80.

Kidd, P., & Morrison, E. F. (1988). The progression of knowledge in nursing: A search for meaning. *Image: Journal of Nursing Scholarship, 20.*

Limandri, B. J. (1982). Book reviews. *Western Journal of Nursing Research, 4*(1), 105-106.

Malinski, V. M. (1990). Three perspectives on a scholarly issue. *Nursing Science Quarterly, 3,* 49-50.

Moch, S. D., & Diemert, C. A. (1987). Health promotion within the nursing environment. *Nursing Administration Quarterly, 11*(3), 9-12.

Moody, L. (1990). Advancing nursing science through research, Vols. 1 & 2. Newbury Park, CA: Sage.

Pearson, B. D. (1987). Pain control: An experiment with imagery. *Geriatric Nursing, 8*(1), 28-30.

Perry, J. (1985). Has the discipline of nursing developed to the stage where nurses do think nursing? *Journal of Advanced Nursing, 10*(1), 31-37.

Phillips, J. R. (1990). Guest editorial: New methods of research: Beyond the shadows of nursing science. *Nursing Science Quarterly, 3,* 1-2.

Ray, M. A. (1987). Technological caring: A new model in critical care. *Dimensions of Critical Care Nursing, 6*(3), 166-173.

Ray, M. A. (1990). Critical reflective analysis of Parse's and Newman's research methodologies. *Nursing Science Quarterly, 3,* 44-46.

Reed, P. G. (1986). Religiousness among terminally ill and healthy adults. *Research in Nursing and Health, 9*(1), 35-41.

Reed, P. G. (1987). Constructing a conceptual framework for psychosocial nursing. *Journal of Psychosocial Nursing and Mental Health Services, 25*(2), 24-28.

Ruffingrahal, M. A. (1985). Qualitative methods in community analysis. *Public Health Nursing, 2,* 130-137.

Sarter, B. (1987). Evolutionary idealism: A philosophical foundation for holistic nursing theory. *Advances in Nursing Science, 9,* 1-9.

Sarter, B. (1988). Philosophical sources of nursing theory. *Nursing Science Quarterly, 1,* 52-59.

Smith, M. J. (1984). Transformation: A key to shaping nursing. *Image, 16*(1), 28-30.

Smith, M. C. (1990). Nursing's unique focus on health promotion. *Nursing Science Quarterly, 3,* 105-106.

Smith, M. C. (1990). Pattern in nursing practice. *Nursing Science Quarterly, 3,* 57-59.

Thompson, J. L. (1985). Practical discourse in nursing: Going beyond empiricism and historicism. *Advances in Nursing Science, 7*(4), 59-71.

Uys, L. R. (1987). Foundational studies in nursing. *Journal of Advanced Nursing, 12*(3), 275-280.

About the Author

Sheila Bunting has spent many years in nursing practice, education, and administration and is presently a doctoral candidate in nursing at Wayne State University in Detroit, Michigan. She received earlier nursing degrees from St. Ambrose College, Davenport, the University of Illinois, and Northern Illinois University. Her clinical area of practice is community health nursing. Her interests and publication topics include feminist and ethical theories and the historical and current interactions of these theories with nursing. Her research pursuits have involved, in addition to nursing ethics, family/friend caregiving to individuals with chronic illnesses. Her dissertation, for which she has been granted a National Research Service Award and received funding from the Michigan Health Care Education and Research Foundation, is a grounded theory study of persons with AIDS and their caregivers.